DASH DIET FOR WOMEN

Introduction to the DASH diet for women who want to lose weight and manage or get rid of hypertension

© Copyright 2020 by EVELYN MOORE All rights reserved.

This document is geared towards providing exact and reliable information in regards to the topic and issue covered. The publication is sold with the idea that the publisher is not required to render accounting, officially permitted, or otherwise, qualified services. If advice is necessary, legal or professional, a practiced individual in the profession should be ordered.

- From a Declaration of Principles which was accepted and approved equally by a Committee of the American Bar Association and a Committee of Publishers and Associations.

In no way is it legal to reproduce, duplicate, or transmit any part of this document in either electronic means or in printed format. Recording of this publication is strictly prohibited and any storage of this document is not allowed unless with written permission from the publisher. All rights reserved.

The information provided herein is stated to be truthful and consistent, in that any liability, in terms of inattention or otherwise, by any usage or abuse of any policies, processes, or directions contained within is the solitary and utter responsibility of the recipient reader. Under no circumstances will any legal responsibility or blame be held against the publisher for any reparation, damages, or monetary loss due to the information herein, either directly or indirectly.

Respective authors own all copyrights not held by the publisher.

The information herein is offered for informational purposes solely, and is universal as so. The presentation of the information is without contract or any type of guarantee assurance.

TABLE OF CONTENTS

Introduction 1

Chapter 1: DASH Breakfast Recipes 4

   1. Tofu Scramble 4

   2. Almond Banana Smoothie 6

   3. Spinach and Mushroom Omelette 7

   4. Eggplant Parmesan 8

   5. Zucchini Stuffed with Italian Sausage 10

   6. Spiced Grilled Salmon 12

   7. DASH Seasoned Rice Mix 13

   8. Cobb Salad (Thai-Style) 14

   9. Asparagus Omelet Tortilla Wrap 15

   10. Banana Pancakes (Whole Wheat) 16

Chapter 2: Main Course 17

   1. Tomato Curried Pork Chops 17

   2. Chicken Thai Pasta 18

   3. Lentil Medley 19

   4. Lemon Salmon with Farro and Caponata 20

   5. Green Bean Tomato Soup 22

   6. Sole Fillet with Mushrooms 23

   7. Egg and Spinach Stuffed Portobello Mushrooms 24

   8. Orzo Pasta with Shrimp and Feta Cheese 25

   9. Pasta with Beef and Pesto 26

10. Pork Roast with Herb and Citrus 27
11. Limed Tilapia Fillets with Pineapple Salsa 29
12. California Quinoa 30
13. Pepper, Tuna, and Mango Kebabs 31
14. Chicken with Cherry Lettuce Wraps 32
15. White Cheddar and Black Bean Frittata 33
16. Cauliflower Steak Curry with Tzatziki Sauce and Red Rice 34
17. Barley Vegetable and Turkey Soup 36
18. Grilled Steak Salad (Southwestern Style) 37
19. Cabbage Rolls 39
20. Pinto Beans Salad with Rice 40

Chapter 3: DASH Desserts 41

1. Grilled Pineapple with Lime and Chili 41
2. Homemade Spicy Almonds 42
3. Rice and Mango Pudding 43
4. Cranberry Blueberry Smoothie 44
5. Peach Raspberry Puff Pancake 45
6. Peach Tart 46
7. Blueberry Apple Cobbler 47
8. Orange Smoothie 49
9. Grilled Angel Food Cake 50
10. Cream and Cookies Shake 51

Chapter 4: DASH Snacks 52

1. Steamed Asparagus with Horseradish Dip 52
2. Mint, Lime, and Grapefruit Yogurt Parfait 53
3. Pita Chips with Hummus Dip 54
4. Almond and Fruit Bites 55

5. Banana Split—DASH Diet Style 56
6. Chai Almond Granola...57
7. Almond Butter and Chocolate Bites 58
8. Hummus and Vegetables Sandwich..59
9. Banana Peanut Butter Cinnamon Toast...60
10. Oat with Peanut Butter Energy Balls..61

Conclusion **62**

INTRODUCTION

The increasing number of people with hypertension has become a source of huge concern worldwide. The number of people who have high blood pressure has more than doubled in the last four decades.

This phenomenon is a source of huge concern since hypertension is linked to other serious health conditions such as stroke, kidney failure, and heart diseases. According to researchers, the increase in the numbers has shifted from European countries to Asian countries [1].

What this and other research [2] tells us is that hypertension is now a global concern. It affects people of any age, nationality, race or creed. High blood pressure is also a huge concern among women.

Cardiovascular disease is a greater health concern for women more than any other disease. According to one study by researchers and medical personnel from Oslo University Hospital [3], hypertension is often underestimated especially in women.

It is actually a very important risk factor. Currently the guidelines for treating hypertension are the same for men and women. However, experts recommend more studies and better guidelines for women since they experience this condition differently compared to men.

In fact, according to one study [4], women who come from middle to low income countries have a higher blood pressure prevalence compared to women who come from countries with a higher income.

Globally, the same study reports, there is a higher use of antihypertensive medication in women compared to men. What this means is that there is a rising number of women who are experiencing high blood pressure.

The good news is that there is a higher awareness of this condition among women than in men. That means they are more likely to take care of themselves and find solutions to better manage their blood pressure.

One of the ways to do just that is to try the DASH diet.

This diet actually provides a number of remarkable benefits especially for women. They include the following:

- ***Decreases the risk of heart disease*** – according to one research, women who do the DASH diet reduce their risk of heart disease as much as 20%. It also lowers their risk for stroke by 29%.
- ***Lowers the risk for diabetes*** – studies show that women who follow a type of DASH diet improve their insulin resistance thus lowering their risk for type 2 diabetes.
- ***Lowers risk for metabolic syndrome*** – the DASH diet also reduces a person's risk for metabolic syndrome up to 81%.

Note that a lot of the heart protective benefits of the DASH diet is attributed by medical experts to the fact that it requires the consumption of a lot of veggies and fruits.

Remember DASH is short for Dietary Approaches to Stop Hypertension. This diet was specifically designed to reduce and prevent hypertension.

Some women may be afraid that this type of diet is another one of those highly restrictive diets out there. Some may even think that it is just another fad diet.

Judging from the evidence and also from my personal experience, it is a diet that can help you manage your weight and your blood pressure. It's not very restrictive at all. You'll be eating plenty of fruits and veggies but you can also have lean meat, and whole grains.

DASH diet recipes are also wonderful. In fact, they are scrumptious. What you may even find surprising is the dessert line—you can still have smoothies and cakes!

This recipe book covers all the bases from breakfast recipes, main courses, desserts, and snacks. I have included all the essential nutritional information along with the prep times for each recipe.

They are very easy to do and a lot of them won't take a lot of your time to prepare. There are some recipes that I have included here that will take some more time to cook but they are absolutely divine and worth the wait and effort.

The DASH diet is rated as one of the best diets for addressing hypertension in women. One report [5] tells us that this diet has a high potency for improving heart health in women.

It is my hope that the recipes in this book will help you get deliciously started on the DASH diet and pave the way to better heart health.

CHAPTER 1:
DASH BREAKFAST RECIPES

1. TOFU SCRAMBLE

Prep Time: 10 minutes
Cook Time: 20 minutes
Serving Size: 1/2 of the dish

INGREDIENTS:

Scramble:

- 8 ounces tofu (extra-firm)
- 2 cups kale (chopped loosely)
- 1/2 red pepper (sliced thinly)
- 1/4 red onion (sliced thinly)
- 2 tablespoons olive oil

Sauce:

- 1/2 teaspoon ground cumin
- 1/2 teaspoon garlic powder
- 1/2 teaspoon sea salt
- 1/4 teaspoon chili powder
- 1/4 teaspoon turmeric
- Water (to thin)

Serving:

- Toast

DIRECTIONS:

1. Pat the tofu to dry using paper towels.
2. In a bowl, combine all the sauce ingredients. Mix well. Add a little water just enough to make it pourable.
3. In a skillet over medium heat, heat up the olive oil. Sautee the red pepper and onion for 5 minutes. Season with pepper and salt.
4. Stir in the kale. Cover for 2 minutes.
5. In a plate, crumble the tofu into bite-sized pieces using a fork.
6. Move the vegetables to one side of the skillet. Put in the tofu on the empty space. Cook for 2 minutes.

7. Pour the sauce over the tofu and the vegetables. Stir everything to mix well. Cook for 7 minutes.
8. Serve with toast.

Nutrition:
Calories: 212 | Carbohydrates: 7.1 g
Fat: 15.1 g | Protein: 16.4 g

2. ALMOND BANANA SMOOTHIE

Prep Time: 3 minutes
Cook Time: 2 minutes
Serving Size: 1 glass

INGREDIENTS:

- 1/2 cup almond milk
- 1 large banana (one-inch slices, frozen)
- 2 spoonfuls flax seed
- 1 heaping spoonful almond butter
- Tiny drop of almond extract
- Drizzle of maple syrup

DIRECTIONS:

1. In a blender, put in all the ingredients.
2. Blend until smooth.
3. Transfer into a glass. Serve.

Nutrition:
Calories: 376 | Carbohydrates: 48.3 g
Fat: 19.4 g | Protein: 9.2 g

3. SPINACH AND MUSHROOM OMELETTE

Prep Time: 3 minutes
Cook Time: 15 minutes
Serving Size: 1 omelet

INGREDIENTS:

- 1 1/2 cup fresh spinach (chopped)
- 1/4 cup red onion (sliced)
- 5 baby bella mushrooms (sliced)
- 1 ounce goat cheese (crumbled)
- 2 egg whites
- 1 whole egg
- 1 tablespoon olive oil
- Cooking spray
- Green onions (diced, for garnish)

DIRECTIONS:

1. In a skillet over medium heat, heat the olive oil. Sautee the red onions for 3 minutes.
2. Add the mushrooms. Sautee for 5 minutes.
3. Add the spinach. Sautee for 2 minutes. Season with pepper and salt. Set aside.
4. In another skillet over medium heat, spray with cooking spray.
5. In a bowl, put in the egg whites and whole egg. Whisk.
6. Pour the egg mixture on the heated skillet. Let it sit for a minute. Tilt the skillet to get the runny eggs in the center to cook on the sides. Do this until there are no more runny eggs.
7. Put the spinach-mushroom mixture and goat cheese on top of a side of the omelet. Fold the other side over the toppings. Cook for half a minute.
8. Serve with green onions as garnish.

Nutrition:
Calories: 412 | Carbohydrates: 18 g
Fat: 29 g | Protein: 25 g

4. EGGPLANT PARMESAN

Prep Time: 10 minutes
Cook Time: 1 hour
Serving Size: 1/6 of the dish

INGREDIENTS:

- 2 1/2 cups tomato sauce
- 1 cup breadcrumbs (fine dry)
- 3/4 cup part-skim mozzarella cheese (grated)
- 1/2 cup Parmesan cheese (freshly grated, divided)
- 1/4 cup fresh basil leaves (slivered)
- 3 egg whites
- 2 eggplants
- 3 tablespoons water
- 1/2 teaspoon freshly ground pepper
- 1/2 teaspoon salt

DIRECTIONS:

1. Preheat oven to 400 degrees Fahrenheit. Grease a baking dish and 2 baking pans with nonstick cooking spray.
2. Slice the eggplants crosswise making 1/4-inch thick slices.
3. In a dish, whisk the water and egg whites until frothy.
4. In another dish, mix well the breadcrumbs, salt, 1/4 cup Parmesan, and pepper.
5. Dip each eggplant slices in the egg white mixture. Coat each slices with the breadcrumb mixture.
6. Arrange the eggplant on the greased baking pans.
7. Bake for 15 minutes. Turn each slice over. Bake for another 15 minutes.
8. In a bowl, mix well the tomato sauce and basil. Pour 1/2 cup of the sauce onto the greased baking dish. Spread evenly.
9. Portion the eggplant slices into two. Arrange the first portion over the sauce on the baking dish. The edges are overlapping slightly.
10. Pour a cup of the tomato sauce over the arranged eggplant slices. Sprinkle half of the mozzarella cheese on top.
11. Layer the second portion of the eggplant slices on top of the

cheese. Pour the rest of the tomato sauce over. Sprinkle with the rest of the Parmesan and mozzarella.
12. Bake for 20 minutes. Serve.

Nutrition:
Calories: 204 | Carbohydrates: 29.2 g
Fat: 5.9 g | Protein: 11.3 g

5. ZUCCHINI STUFFED WITH ITALIAN SAUSAGE

Prep Time: 35 minutes
Cook Time: 20 minutes
Serving Size: 2 stuffed zucchini halves

INGREDIENTS:

- 1 pound Italian turkey sausage (casings removed)
- 6 medium zucchinis
- 2 medium tomatoes (seeded, chopped)
- 1 cup panko bread crumbs
- 3/4 cup part-skim mozzarella cheese (shredded)
- 1/3 cup fresh parsley (minced)
- 1/3 cup Parmesan cheese (grated)
- 2 tablespoons fresh basil (minced)
- 2 tablespoons fresh oregano (minced)
- 1/4 teaspoon pepper
- Fresh parsley (minced, for garnish)

DIRECTIONS:

1. Preheat your oven to 350 degrees Fahrenheit.
2. Cut the zucchinis in half, lengthwise. Scoop out the pulp. Leave 1/4-inch of pulp in the shell. Chop the pulp. Set aside.
3. Microwave the zucchini shells for 3 minutes.
4. In a skillet over medium heat, cook the zucchini pulp and sausage for 8 minutes. Break the sausages into crumbles. Drain the liquid. Turn off the heat.
5. Add in the bread crumbs, tomatoes, herbs, Parmesan cheese, and pepper. Stir to mix.
6. Spoon the mixture into the zucchini shells.
7. Put the stuffed shells into ungreased baking dishes. Cover. Bake for 20 minutes.
8. Uncover. Sprinkle the mozzarella cheese on top. Bake for 8 minutes.
9. Garnish with parsley. Serve.

Nutrition:
Calories: 206 | Carbohydrates: 16 g
Fat: 9 g | Protein: 17 g

6. SPICED GRILLED SALMON

Prep Time: 5 minutes
Cook Time: 15 minutes
Serving Size: 3 ounces of cooked salmon

INGREDIENTS:

- 1 (2 pounds) salmon fillet
- 2 tablespoons packed brown sugar
- 1 tablespoon butter (melted)
- 1 tablespoon soy sauce
- 1 tablespoon olive oil
- 1/2 teaspoon pepper
- 1/2 teaspoon ground mustard
- 1/2 teaspoon garlic powder
- 1/2 teaspoon paprika
- 1/4 teaspoon dill weed
- Dash dried tarragon
- Dash salt
- Dash cayenne pepper

DIRECTIONS:

1. In a bowl, mix all the ingredients except the salmon.
2. Brush the mixture on the salmon.
3. Lightly oil the grill rack on medium heat. Put the salmon skin side down. Grill for 15 minutes.
4. Serve.

Nutrition:
Calories: 256 | Carbohydrates: 5 g
Fat: 17 g | Protein: 20 g

7. DASH SEASONED RICE MIX

Prep Time: 10 minutes
Cook Time: 20 minutes
Serving Size: ½ of the dish

INGREDIENTS:

- 1/2 cup dried vegetable flakes
- 4 cups instant brown rice (uncooked)
- 2 tablespoons dried parsley
- 2 tablespoons low-sodium bouillon granules (chicken-flavored)
- 2 teaspoons dried rosemary (crushed)
- 1 teaspoon garlic powder
- 1 teaspoon dried marjoram
- 1/2 teaspoon ground black pepper

DIRECTIONS:

1. In a bowl, mix together the rice, vegetable flakes, bouillon, rosemary, parsley, garlic powder, marjoram, and pepper.
2. In a saucepan over medium heat, boil 1 cup of water.
3. Stir in a cup of rice mix. Let it boil.
4. Lower heat. Simmer for 5 minutes.
5. Turn off heat. Stir. Cover. Let the cooked rice stand for 5 minutes. Fluff the rice using a fork. Serve.

Nutrition:
Calories: 109 | Carbohydrates: 23 g
Fat: 1 g | Protein: 2 g

8. COBB SALAD (THAI-STYLE)

Prep Time: 10 minutes
Cook Time: 5 minutes
Serving Size: 1/6 of the dish

INGREDIENTS:

- 2 cups rotisserie chicken (shredded)
- 1 cup fresh snow peas (halved)
- 3/4 cup Asian toasted sesame salad dressing
- 1/4 cup fresh cilantro leaves
- 1/2 cup peanuts (unsalted)
- 1 bunch romaine (torn)
- 1 medium carrot (shredded)
- 1 medium ripe avocado (peeled, sliced thinly)
- 1 medium sweet red pepper (julienned)
- 3 large hard-boiled eggs (chopped coarsely)
- 2 tablespoons creamy peanut butter

DIRECTIONS:

1. In a serving platter, arrange the romaine in a single layer. Top with chicken, avocado, eggs, peanuts, and vegetables. Garnish with cilantro.
2. In a bowl, whisk the peanut butter and salad dressing until smooth.
3. Serve the salad with the dressing on the side.

Nutrition:
Calories: 382 | Carbohydrates: 18 g
Fat: 25 g | Protein: 23 g

9. ASPARAGUS OMELET TORTILLA WRAP

Prep Time: 5 minutes
Cook Time: 15 minutes
Serving Size: 1 tortilla wrap

INGREDIENTS:

- 4 fresh asparagus spears (trimmed, sliced)
- 1 8-inch whole wheat tortilla (warmed)
- 1 green onion (chopped)
- 2 large egg whites
- 1 large egg
- 1 tablespoon milk (fat-free)
- 2 teaspoons Parmesan cheese (grated)
- 1 teaspoon butter
- 1/8 teaspoon pepper

DIRECTIONS:

1. In a bowl, whisk the egg whites, whole egg, milk, cheese, and pepper.
2. In a non-stick skillet over medium heat, spritz some cooking spray. Cook the asparagus for 4 minutes. Set aside.
3. In the same skillet over medium heat, melt the butter. Pour the egg mixture. Let it sit for a minute. Tilt the skillet to let the runny eggs to the edges to set. Do this until there are no more runny eggs.
4. Place the asparagus and green onions on one side of the omelet. Fold the other side over the topping.
5. Serve the omelet in a tortilla wrap.

Nutrition:
Calories: 319 | *Carbohydrates*: 28 g
Fat: 13 g | *Protein:* 21 g

10. BANANA PANCAKES (WHOLE WHEAT)

Prep Time: 10 minutes
Cook Time: 20 minutes
Serving Size: 2 pancakes

INGREDIENTS:

- 2 cups milk (fat-free)
- 1 cup all-purpose flour
- 1 cup whole wheat flour
- 2/3 cup ripe banana (mashed)
- 2 large eggs
- 1 tablespoon maple syrup
- 1 tablespoon olive oil
- 4 teaspoons baking powder
- 1/2 teaspoon salt
- 1 teaspoon ground cinnamon
- 1/2 teaspoon vanilla extract
- Sliced bananas and more maple syrup (for serving)

DIRECTIONS:

1. In a bowl, whisk together the wheat flour, all-purpose flour, baking powder, cinnamon, and salt.
2. In another bowl, whisk together the milk, eggs, oil, mashed banana, vanilla, and maple syrup. Stir in the flour mixture until a batter is formed.
3. Coat a griddle with cooking spray. Preheat it over medium heat.
4. Scoop 1/4 cup of batter. Pour it on the griddle. Cook the pancake until golden brown on each side.
5. Serve with sliced bananas and maple syrup.

Nutrition:
Calories: 186 | *Carbohydrates*: 32 g
Fat: 4 g | *Protein:* 7 g

CHAPTER 2:
MAIN COURSE

1. TOMATO CURRIED PORK CHOPS

Prep Time: 15 minutes
Cook Time: 25 minutes
Serving Size: 2/3 cup rice, 3/4 cup tomato mixture, and 1 pork chop

INGREDIENTS:

- 6 pork loin chops (boneless)
- 1 28-ounce can whole tomatoes (undrained)
- 3 medium apples (sliced thinly)
- 1 small onion (chopped finely)
- 4 cups brown rice (cooked, still hot)
- 4 teaspoons sugar
- 4 teaspoons butter (divided)
- 2 teaspoons curry powder
- 1/2 teaspoon chili powder
- 1/2 teaspoon salt

DIRECTIONS:

1. In a stockpot over medium heat, melt 2 teaspoons of butter. Brown the pork chops by batch. Set aside.
2. In the same stockpot over medium heat, melt the rest of the butter. Sautee onion for 3 minutes.
3. Stir in the tomatoes, apples, salt, sugar, curry powder, and chili powder. Let it boil with regular stirring to break the tomatoes.
4. Put the pork chops back into the stockpot. Lower the heat. Let the mixture simmer for 5 minutes.
5. Flip the pork chops. Simmer for 5 minutes more. Turn off the heat.
6. Let the dish stand for 5 minutes before serving.
7. Serve with rice.

Nutrition:
Calories: 478 | Carbohydrates: 50 g
Fat: 14 g | Protein: 38 g

2. CHICKEN THAI PASTA

Prep Time: 10 minutes
Cook Time: 20 minutes
Serving Size: 1 1/3 cups

INGREDIENTS:

- 1 10-ounce pack fresh sugar snap peas (trimmed, diagonal thin strip slices)
- 6 ounces whole wheat spaghetti (uncooked)
- 2 cups cooked chicken (shredded)
- 2 cups carrots (julienned)
- 1 cup Thai peanut sauce
- 2 teaspoons canola oil
- 1 medium cucumber (halved lengthwise, seeded, diagonal slices)
- Fresh cilantro (chopped, for garnish)

DIRECTIONS:

1. Cook the spaghetti according to package instructions.
2. In a skillet over medium heat, heat up the oil. Stir fry the carrots and snap peas for 8 minutes.
3. Add the peanut sauce, chicken, and spaghetti. Toss to combine. Cook until heated through.
4. Put on a plate. Garnish with cilantro and cucumber.

Nutrition:
Calories: 403 | Carbohydrates: 43 g
Fat: 15 g | Protein: 25 g

3. LENTIL MEDLEY

Prep Time: 15 minutes
Cook Time: 25 minutes
Serving Size: 1 1/4 cups

INGREDIENTS:

- 4 cups fresh baby spinach (chopped)
- 2 cups fresh mushrooms (sliced)
- 2 cups water
- 1 cup dried lentils (rinsed)
- 1 cup feta cheese (crumbled)
- 1/2 cup rice vinegar
- 1/2 cup soft sun-dried tomato halves (not packed in oil, chopped)
- 1/4 cup fresh mint (minced)
- 1 medium zucchini (cubed)
- 1 small red onion (chopped)
- 1 medium cucumber (cubed)
- 3 tablespoons olive oil
- 1 teaspoon dried basil
- 2 teaspoons honey
- 1 teaspoon dried oregano

DIRECTIONS:

1. In a saucepan over medium heat, put the water and lentils. Bring to a boil.
2. Lower the heat. Simmer for 25 minutes. Drain. Rinse with cold water.
3. Place the lentils in a bowl. Add the cucumber, mushrooms, onion, zucchini, and tomatoes. Mix.
4. In another bowl, whisk the oil, vinegar, honey, mint, oregano, and basil. Drizzle the mixture over the lentil mixture. Toss.
5. Add the spinach and cheese. Toss. Serve.

Nutrition:
Calories: 225 | Carbohydrates: 29 g
Fat: 8 g | Protein: 10 g

4. LEMON SALMON WITH FARRO AND CAPONATA

Prep Time: 10 minutes
Cook Time: 40 minutes
Serving Size: 3 ounces salmon, 1/2 cup farro, and 1 cup vegetables

INGREDIENTS:

- 1 1/4 pounds wild salmon (cut into 4 portions)
- 2 cups water
- 1 1/2 cups cherry tomatoes
- 2/3 cup farro
- 1 red bell pepper (1-inch pieces)
- 1 medium eggplant (1 inch cubes)
- 1 small onion (1-inch pieces)
- 1 summer squash (1-inch pieces)
- 3 tablespoons extra-virgin olive oil
- 1 tablespoon red-wine vinegar
- 2 tablespoons capers (rinsed, chopped)
- 1 teaspoon lemon zest
- 2 teaspoons honey
- 3/4 teaspoon salt (divided)
- 1/2 teaspoon Italian seasoning
- 1/2 teaspoon ground pepper (divided)
- Lemon wedges (for serving)

DIRECTIONS:

1. Position the racks in the lower and upper thirds of your oven. Preheat to 450 degrees Fahrenheit. Line two rimmed baking tray with foil. Grease them with cooking spray.
2. In a saucepan over medium heat, boil the farro in water. Lower the heat. Cover. Simmer for 30 minutes. Drain any excess liquid.
3. In a bowl, toss the bell pepper, eggplant, onion, squash, 1/2 teaspoon salt, tomatoes, and 1/4 teaspoon pepper. Divide the mixture between the two lined baking trays.
4. Roast for 25 minutes stirring halfway. Put them back into the bowl. Mix in the vinegar, capers, and honey.
5. Season the salmon with Italian seasoning, lemon zest, and the rest of the pepper and salt.

6. Put the salmon on one of the baking trays. Roast for 10 minutes.
7. Serve the salmon with vegetable caponata, farro, and lemon wedges.

Nutrition:
Calories: 256 | Carbohydrates: 5 g
Fat: 17 g | Protein: 20 g

5. GREEN BEAN TOMATO SOUP

Prep Time: 10 minutes
Cook Time: 35 minutes
Serving Size: 1 cup

INGREDIENTS:

- 1 pound fresh green beans (1-inch pieces)
- 1 garlic clove (minced)
- 6 cups vegetable broth (reduced-sodium)
- 3 cups fresh tomatoes (diced)
- 1 cup carrots (chopped)
- 1 cup onion (chopped)
- 1/4 cup fresh basil (minced)
- 2 teaspoons butter
- 1/4 teaspoon pepper
- 1/2 teaspoon salt

DIRECTIONS:

1. In a saucepan over medium heat, melt the butter. Sautee the onion and carrots for 5 minutes.
2. Add the broth, garlic, and beans. Stir. Bring to a boil. Lower the heat. Cover. Simmer for 20 minutes.
3. Add the basil, tomatoes, pepper, and salt. Cover. Simmer for 5 minutes more. Serve.

Nutrition:
Calories: 58 | Carbohydrates: 10 g
Fat: 1 g | Protein: 4 g

6. SOLE FILLET WITH MUSHROOMS

Prep Time: 10 minutes
Cook Time: 15 minutes
Serving Size: 1 sole fillet and 1/4 part of the vegetables

INGREDIENTS:

- 2 cups fresh mushrooms (sliced)
- 4 4-ounce sole fillets
- 2 garlic cloves (minced)
- 2 green onions (sliced thinly)
- 1 medium tomato (chopped)
- 2 tablespoons butter
- 1/4 teaspoon lemon-pepper seasoning
- 1/4 teaspoon paprika
- 1/8 teaspoon cayenne pepper

DIRECTIONS:

1. In a skillet over medium heat, melt the butter. Cook the mushrooms until tender. Stir in the garlic. Cook for a minute more.
2. Put the sole fillets on top of the mushrooms. Season with cayenne, lemon-pepper, and paprika.
3. Cover. Cook for 10 minutes. Garnish with green onions and tomatoes. Serve.

Nutrition:
Calories: 174 | Carbohydrates: 4 g
Fat: 7 g | Protein: 23 g

7. EGG AND SPINACH STUFFED PORTOBELLO MUSHROOMS

Prep Time: 10 minutes
Cook Time: 15 minutes
Serving Size: 1 stuffed mushroom

INGREDIENTS:

- 1 cup fresh baby spinach
- 1/4 cup feta cheese (crumbled)
- 2 large portobello mushrooms (stemmed)
- 1/2 teaspoon olive oil
- 1/8 teaspoon garlic salt
- 1/8 teaspoon salt
- 1/8 teaspoon pepper
- 2 large eggs
- 1 small onion (chopped)
- Cooking spray
- Fresh basil (minced, for garnish)

DIRECTIONS:

1. Preheat oven to 425 degrees Fahrenheit.
2. Spray the mushrooms with cooking spray. Put them stem side up on a baking pan. Season with pepper and garlic salt.
3. Bake for 10 minutes.
4. In a skillet over medium heat, heat the oil. Sautee the onion for 3 minutes. Stir in the spinach. Cook until wilted.
5. In a bowl, whisk the salt and eggs. Stir in the mixture onto the skillet. Cook until the eggs have set.
6. Spoon the spinach mixture into the mushrooms. Garnish with basil and cheese. Serve.

Nutrition:
Calories: 126 | Carbohydrates: 10 g
Fat: 5 g | Protein: 11 g

8. ORZO PASTA WITH SHRIMP AND FETA CHEESE

Prep Time: 10 minutes
Cook Time: 15 minutes
Serving Size: 1 cup

INGREDIENTS:

- 1 1/4 pounds shrimp (uncooked, peeled, deveined)
- 1 1/4 cups whole wheat orzo pasta (uncooked)
- 1/2 cup feta cheese (crumbled)
- 2 medium tomatoes (chopped)
- 2 garlic cloves (minced)
- 2 tablespoons olive oil
- 2 tablespoons fresh cilantro (minced)
- 2 tablespoons lemon juice
- 1/4 teaspoon pepper

DIRECTIONS:

1. Cook the orzo pasta according to package instructions. Drain.
2. In a skillet over medium heat, heat the oil. Sautee the garlic for a minute. Stir in the tomatoes and lemon juice. Let it boil.
3. Stir in the shrimp. Lower the heat. Simmer for 5 minutes.
4. Add the orzo pasta, pepper, and cilantro into the simmering shrimp. Cook until heated through. Garnish with feta cheese. Serve.

Nutrition:
Calories: 406 | Carbohydrates: 40 g
Fat: 12 g | Protein: 33 g

9. PASTA WITH BEEF AND PESTO

Prep Time: 10 minutes
Cook Time: 25 minutes
Serving Size: 1/4 part of the dish

INGREDIENTS:

- 2 cups grape tomatoes (halved)
- 2 cups whole wheat penne pasta (uncooked)
- 1/3 cup prepared pesto
- 1/4 cup Gorgonzola cheese (crumbled)
- 1/4 cup California Walnuts (chopped)
- 5 ounces fresh baby spinach (chopped coarsely)
- 2 6-ounce beef tenderloin steaks
- 1/4 teaspoon pepper
- 1/4 teaspoon salt

DIRECTIONS:

1. Cook the penne pasta according to package instructions. Drain.
2. Season the beef steaks with pepper and salt. Grill the steaks over medium heat to your desired doneness.
3. Put the pasta in a bowl. Add the spinach, pesto, tomatoes, and walnuts. Toss.
4. Slice the beef steak thinly. Serve the pasta with the beef slices. Garnish with cheese.

Nutrition:
Calories: 532 | Carbohydrates: 49 g
Fat: 22 g | Protein: 35 g

10. PORK ROAST WITH HERB AND CITRUS

Prep Time: 25 hours
Cook Time: 5 hours
Serving Size: 5 ounces pork and 2 tablespoons gravy

INGREDIENTS:

- 1 4-pound pork sirloin roast (boneless)
- 2 medium onions (thin wedges)
- 1 cup + 3 tablespoons orange juice (divided)
- 3 tablespoons cornstarch
- 1 tablespoon white grapefruit juice
- 1 tablespoon sugar
- 1 tablespoon soy sauce (reduced-sodium)
- 1 tablespoon steak sauce
- 1 teaspoon dried oregano
- 1 teaspoon orange zest (grated)
- 1/2 teaspoon pepper
- 1/2 teaspoon ground ginger
- 1/2 teaspoon salt

DIRECTIONS:

1. Slice the pork roast in halve.
2. In a bowl, mix together the pepper, ginger, and oregano. Rub the mixture all over the pork.
3. In a greased skillet over medium heat, brown the pork roast on each side.
4. Put the browned pork roast in a slow cooker.
5. Add the onions.
6. In a bowl, mix together the soy sauce, steak sauce, grapefruit juice, sugar, and 1 cup of orange juice. Pour the mixture over the pork roast.
7. Cover the pot. Cook for 5 hours on low setting.
8. Transfer the onions and pork meat to a platter. Set aside.
9. Remove the fat from the cooking juices. Pour the cooking juices into a saucepan over medium heat.
10. Stir in the salt and orange zest. Let it boil.

11. In a bowl, mix well the remaining orange juice and cornstarch. Gradually pour the mixture into the boiling mixture. Stir. Cook until thickened.
12. Serve the pork with the gravy.

Nutrition:
Calories: 289 | Carbohydrates: 13 g
Fat: 10 g | Protein: 35 g

11. LIMED TILAPIA FILLETS WITH PINEAPPLE SALSA

Prep Time: 5 minutes
Cook Time: 15 minutes
Serving Size: 1 tilapia fillet and 1/4 cup pineapple salsa

INGREDIENTS:

- 8 4-ounce tilapia fillets
- 2 cups fresh pineapple (cubed)
- 1/4 cup fresh cilantro (minced)
- 1/4 cup green pepper (chopped finely)
- 1 tablespoon canola oil
- 4 teaspoons + 2 tablespoons lime juice (divided)
- 1/8 teaspoon pepper
- 1/8 teaspoon + 1/4 teaspoon salt (divided)
- 2 green onions (chopped)
- Dash cayenne pepper

DIRECTIONS:

1. In a bowl, mix together the cayenne, 1/8 teaspoon salt, 4 teaspoons lime juice, cilantro, green pepper, green onions, and pineapple. Refrigerate until serving.
2. In another bowl, mix together the remaining lime juice and oil. Drizzle the mixture over the tilapia fillets. Season with the remaining salt and pepper.
3. Coat the grill rack with cooking oil. Grill the fish over medium heat for 3 minutes each side.
4. Serve the fish with the chilled salsa.

Nutrition:
Calories: 131 | Carbohydrates: 6 g
Fat: 3 g | Protein: 21 g

12. CALIFORNIA QUINOA

Prep Time: 10 minutes
Cook Time: 20 minutes
Serving Size: 1 cup

INGREDIENTS:

- 2 cups water
- 1 cup quinoa (rinsed, drained)
- 1/2 cup feta cheese (crumbled)
- 3/4 cup canned chickpeas (rinsed, drained)
- 1/4 cup Greek olives (chopped finely)
- 2 garlic cloves (minced)
- 1 medium tomato (chopped finely)
- 1 medium zucchini (chopped)
- 2 tablespoons fresh basil (minced)
- 1 tablespoon olive oil
- 1/4 teaspoon pepper

DIRECTIONS:

1. In a saucepan over medium heat, heat the oil. Stir in the garlic and quinoa for 3 minutes.
2. Add the water and zucchini. Stir. Bring to a boil.
3. Lower the heat. Cover. Simmer for 15 minutes.
4. Stir in the rest of the ingredients. Cook until heated through. Serve.

Nutrition:
Calories: 310 | Carbohydrates: 42 g
Fat: 11 g | Protein: 11 g

13. PEPPER, TUNA, AND MANGO KEBABS

Prep Time: 10 minutes
Cook Time: 20 minutes
Serving Size: 1 kebab

INGREDIENTS:

- 1 pound tuna steaks (1-inch cubes)
- 1/2 cup frozen corn (thawed)
- 1 jalapeno pepper (seeded, chopped)
- 1 medium mango (peeled, 1-inch cubes)
- 4 green onions (chopped)
- 2 large sweet red peppers (2 x 1-inch pieces)
- 2 tablespoons lime juice
- 2 tablespoons fresh parsley (chopped coarsely)
- 1 teaspoon pepper (coarsely ground)

DIRECTIONS:

1. In a bowl, mix together the corn, green onions, jalapeno, parsley, and lime juice. Set aside.
2. Rub the pepper on the tuna. Prepare 4 skewers. Alternately thread on each skewer the mango, tuna, and red peppers.
3. Grease the grill rack. Grill the kebabs on medium heat for 12 minutes with occasional turning.
4. Serve the kebabs with salsa.

Nutrition:
Calories: 205 | Carbohydrates: 20 g
Fat: 2 g | Protein: 29 g

14. CHICKEN WITH CHERRY LETTUCE WRAPS

Prep Time: 10 minutes
Cook Time: 15 minutes
Serving Size: 2 filled lettuce wraps

INGREDIENTS:

- 3/4 pound chicken breasts (boneless, skinless, 3/4-inch cubes)
- 8 Boston lettuce leaves
- 4 green onions (chopped)
- 1 1/4 cups fresh sweet cherries (pitted, coarsely chopped)
- 1 1/2 cups carrots (shredded)
- 1/3 cup almonds (coarsely chopped)
- 2 tablespoons teriyaki sauce (reduced-sodium)
- 2 tablespoons rice vinegar
- 1 tablespoon honey
- 2 teaspoons olive oil
- 1 teaspoon ground ginger
- 1/4 teaspoon pepper
- 1/4 teaspoon salt

DIRECTIONS:

1. Season the chicken breasts with pepper, salt, and ginger.
2. In a skillet over medium heat, heat the oil. Stir in the chicken. Cook for 5 minutes.
3. Turn off the heat. Stir in the cherries, carrots, almonds, and green onions.
4. In a bowl, mix well the honey, teriyaki sauce, and vinegar. Stir the mixture into the chicken and vegetables.
5. Divide the mixture among the lettuce wraps. Secure the filling. Serve.

Nutrition:
Calories: 257 | Carbohydrates: 22 g
Fat: 10 g | Protein: 21 g

15. WHITE CHEDDAR AND BLACK BEAN FRITTATA

Prep Time: 20 minutes
Cook Time: 15 minutes
Serving Size: 1 wedge

INGREDIENTS:

- 1 cup canned black beans (rinsed, drained)
- 1/3 cup sweet red pepper (chopped finely)
- 1/3 cup green pepper (chopped finely)
- 1/2 cup white cheddar cheese (shredded)
- 1/4 cup salsa
- 3 large egg whites
- 6 large eggs
- 2 garlic cloves (minced)
- 3 green onions (chopped finely)
- 1 tablespoon fresh parsley (minced)
- 1 tablespoon olive oil
- 1/4 teaspoon pepper
- 1/4 teaspoon salt

DIRECTIONS:

1. Preheat broiler.
2. In a bowl, whisk well the whole eggs, egg whites, salsa, parsley, salt, and pepper.
3. In an oven-proof skillet over medium heat, heat the oil. Sautee the green onions and peppers for 4 minutes.
4. Stir in the garlic. Cook for a minute.
5. Stir in the beans. Lower the heat. Stir in the egg mixture. Cook until the eggs are almost set. Top with cheese.
6. Broil for 4 minutes about 4 inches from heat.
7. Let it stand for 5 minutes. Slice into 6 wedges. Serve.

Nutrition:
Calories: 183 | Carbohydrates: 9 g
Fat: 10 g | Protein: 13 g

16. CAULIFLOWER STEAK CURRY WITH TZATZIKI SAUCE AND RED RICE

Prep Time: 30 minutes
Cook Time: 30 minutes
Serving Size: 1 cauliflower steak, 3/4 cup rice, and 1/4 cup tzatziki sauce

INGREDIENTS:

Tzatziki Sauce:

- 1/4 cup sour cream
- 3/4 cup plain Greek yogurt (nonfat)
- 1 clove garlic (minced)
- 1 tablespoon lemon juice
- 1/2 medium cucumber (seeded, grated)
- 1/2 teaspoon kosher salt

Cauliflower Steaks and Rice:

- 1/3 cup extra-virgin olive oil
- 1 cup red rice
- 2 tablespoons fresh cilantro (chopped)
- 1 tablespoon lemon juice
- 2 medium heads cauliflower
- 1/2 teaspoon kosher salt
- 2 teaspoons curry powder

DIRECTIONS:

Tzatziki Sauce:

1. In a bowl, whisk the sour cream, yogurt, garlic, lemon juice, and salt until smooth. Fold in the cucumber. Chill in the fridge.

Cauliflower and Rice:

1. Preheat oven to 450 degrees Fahrenheit. Line a rimmed baking tray with foil.
2. Cook rice according to package instructions. Keep warm.
3. In a bowl, whisk well the lemon juice, oil, salt, and curry powder.
4. Discard the outer leaves of the cauliflower. Keep the stems intact.
5. Make 4 cauliflower steaks. They should be 1-inch thick slices from the center of each cauliflower head down to the stem.

6. Cut the rest of the cauliflower into 3/4-inch florets.
7. Place the steaks and florets on the lined baking tray in a single layer. Brush all sides of the cauliflower with the curry mixture.
8. Roast for 35 minutes turning halfway.
9. Store 6 tablespoons of tzatziki sauce and florets in the fridge for another recipe.
10. Equally divide the cooked rice among 4 plates. Top each rice with a steak, 1/4 cup of tzatziki sauce. Garnish with cilantro. Serve.

Nutrition:
Calories: 410 | Carbohydrates: 48.5 g
Fat: 21.3 g | Protein: 10.3 g

17. BARLEY VEGETABLE AND TURKEY SOUP

Prep Time: 5 minutes
Cook Time: 25 minutes
Serving Size: 1 1/3 cups

INGREDIENTS:

- 6 cups chicken broth (reduced-sodium)
- 2 cups fresh baby spinach
- 2 cups cooked turkey breast (cubed)
- 2/3 cup quick-cooking barley
- 1 medium onion (chopped)
- 5 medium carrots (chopped)
- 1 tablespoon canola oil
- 1/2 teaspoon pepper

DIRECTIONS:

1. In a saucepan over medium heat, heat the oil. Sautee the onion and carrots for 5 minutes.
2. Stir in the broth and barley. Bring to a boil.
3. Lower the heat. Cover. Simmer for 15 minutes.
4. Add the spinach, turkey, and pepper. Stir. Cook until heated through. Serve.

Nutrition:
Calories: 208 | Carbohydrates: 23 g
Fat: 4 g | Protein: 21 g

18. GRILLED STEAK SALAD (SOUTHWESTERN STYLE)

Prep Time: 25 minutes
Cook Time: 20 minutes
Serving Size: 2 ounces beef and 2 cups pasta mixture

INGREDIENTS:

- 1 3/4-pound beef top sirloin steak (1 inch thick)
- 2 large ears sweet corn (husks removed)
- 3 poblano peppers (halved, seeded)
- 1 large sweet onion (1/2-inch rings)
- 2 large tomatoes
- 2 cups multigrain bow tie pasta (uncooked)
- 1 tablespoon olive oil
- 1/4 teaspoon ground cumin
- 1/4 teaspoon salt
- 1/4 teaspoon pepper

Dressing:

- 1/3 cup fresh cilantro (chopped)
- 1/4 cup lime juice
- 1/4 teaspoon salt
- 1 tablespoon olive oil
- 1/4 teaspoon pepper
- 1/4 teaspoon ground cumin

DIRECTIONS:

1. Rub the steak with pepper, cumin, and salt.
2. Brush oil on the onion, corn, and poblano peppers.
3. Grill the steak to your desired doneness over medium heat.
4. Grill the oiled vegetables for 10 minutes with occasional turning.
5. Cook the pasta according to package instructions. Drain.
6. Chop the tomatoes, peppers, and onion. Remove the corn from the cob. Put them all in a bowl.
7. In another bowl, whisk together the oil, lime juice, cumin, salt, and pepper. Stir in the cilantro.
8. Add the pasta into the chopped vegetables. Pour the dressing over. Toss.
9. Thinly slice the steak. Add to the salad. Serve.

Nutrition:
Calories: 456 | Carbohydrates: 58 g
Fat: 13 g | Protein: 30 g

19. CABBAGE ROLLS

Prep Time: 15 minutes
Cook Time: 20 minutes
Serving Size: 1 1/3 cups and 2/3 cup rice

INGREDIENTS:

- 1 28-ounce can whole plum tomatoes (undrained)
- 1 8-ounce can tomato sauce
- 1 pound extra-lean ground beef (95% lean)
- 1 large onion (chopped)
- 1 medium green pepper (thin strips)
- 1 small head cabbage (sliced thinly)
- 4 cups brown rice (hot cooked)
- 2 tablespoons cider vinegar
- 1 tablespoon brown sugar
- 1 teaspoon dried thyme (seasoning)
- 1 teaspoon dried oregano (seasoning)
- 1/2 teaspoon pepper (seasoning)

DIRECTIONS:

1. Drain the tomatoes. Set aside the liquid. Chop the tomatoes coarsely.
2. In a skillet over medium heat, cook the onion and beef for 8 minutes.
3. Add in the vinegar, tomato sauce, seasonings, brown sugar, tomatoes, and reserved liquid.
4. Stir in the cabbage and pepper. Cover. Cook for 6 minutes with occasional stirring. Uncover. Cook for another 8 minutes. Serve with rice.

Nutrition:
Calories: 332 | Carbohydrates: 50 g
Fat: 5 g | Protein: 22 g

20. PINTO BEANS SALAD WITH RICE

Prep Time: 10 minutes
Cook Time: 20 minutes
Serving Size: 1/4 part of the dish

INGREDIENTS:

- 1 8.8-ounce package ready-to-serve brown rice
- 1 15-ounce can pinto beans (rinsed, drained)
- 1 4-ounce can green chilies (chopped)
- 1 cup frozen corn
- 1/4 cup fresh cilantro (chopped)
- 1/2 cup salsa
- 1/4 cup cheddar cheese (shredded finely)
- 1 tablespoon olive oil
- 1 1/2 teaspoons ground cumin
- 1 1/2 teaspoons chili powder
- 1 small onion (chopped)
- 1 bunch romaine (4 wedges)
- 2 garlic cloves (minced)

DIRECTIONS:

1. In a skillet over medium heat, heat the oil. Sautee the onion and corn for 5 minutes.
2. Add the cumin, chili powder, and garlic. Sautee for 1 minute more.
3. Add the cilantro, salsa, green chilies, rice, and pinto beans. Cook until heated through with occasional stirring.
4. Put the romaine wedges in a bowl. Pour the pinto bean mixture over the wedges. Garnish with cheese. Serve.

Nutrition:
Calories: 331 | Carbohydrates: 50 g
Fat: 8 g | Protein: 12 g

CHAPTER 3:
DASH DESSERTS

1. GRILLED PINEAPPLE WITH LIME AND CHILI

Prep Time: 5 minutes
Cook Time: 10 minutes
Serving Size: 1 pineapple wedge

INGREDIENTS:

- 3 tablespoons brown sugar
- 1 fresh pineapple
- 1 tablespoon olive oil
- 1 tablespoon lime juice
- 1 1/2 teaspoons chili powder
- 1 tablespoon honey
- Dash salt

DIRECTIONS:

1. Peel the pineapple. Remove the eyes. Slice into 6 wedges. Remove the core.
2. In a bowl, mix well all the ingredients except for the pineapple. Brush half of the glaze on all sides of the pineapple wedges.
3. Grill the pineapple over medium heat for 4 minutes per side with occasional basting with the other half of the glaze. Serve.

Nutrition:
Calories: 97 | Carbohydrates: 20 g
Fat: 2 g | Protein: 1 g

2. HOMEMADE SPICY ALMONDS

Prep Time: 10 minutes
Cook Time: 30 minutes
Serving Size: 1/4 cup

INGREDIENTS:

- 2 1/2 cups almonds (unblanched)
- 1 tablespoon sugar
- 1 large egg white (room temperature)
- 1 1/2 teaspoons kosher salt
- 1/2 teaspoon ground cinnamon
- 1 teaspoon paprika
- 1/2 teaspoon ground cumin
- 1/4 teaspoon cayenne pepper
- 1/2 teaspoon ground coriander

DIRECTIONS:

1. Preheat oven to 325 degrees Fahrenheit. Grease a baking pan.
2. In a bowl, mix well the sugar, kosher salt, paprika, cinnamon, cumin, coriander, and cayenne.
3. In another bowl, whisk well the egg white until foamy. Put the almonds. Toss.
4. Sprinkle the spice mixture over. Toss.
5. Spread out the almonds on the greased baking pan. Bake for 30 minutes with stirring on a 10-minute interval.
6. Let the almonds cool on a wax paper. Serve.

Nutrition:
Calories: 230 | Carbohydrates: 9 g
Fat: 20 g | Protein: 8 g

3. RICE AND MANGO PUDDING

Prep Time: 5 minutes
Cook Time: 50 minutes
Serving Size: 1 cup

INGREDIENTS:

- 2 cups water
- 1 cup long grain brown rice (uncooked)
- 1 cup vanilla soy milk
- 2 tablespoons sugar
- 1 medium ripe mango
- 1 teaspoon vanilla extract
- 1/2 teaspoon ground cinnamon
- 1/4 teaspoon salt

DIRECTIONS:

1. In a saucepan over medium heat, bring salt and water to a boil. Stir in the rice.
2. Lower the heat. Cover. Simmer for 40 minutes.
3. Peel the mango. Slice it. Mash the mango slices using a fork.
4. Add the mashed mango, milk, cinnamon, and sugar into the rice. Stir. Cook for 15 minutes more with occasional stirring.
5. Turn off the heat. Stir in the vanilla. Serve.

Nutrition:
Calories: 275 | Carbohydrates: 58 g
Fat: 3 g | Protein: 6 g

4. CRANBERRY BLUEBERRY SMOOTHIE

Prep Time: 5 minutes
Cook Time: 0 minutes
Serving Size: 2 cups

INGREDIENTS:

- 1 cup frozen blueberries
- 1 cup low-fat plain kefir
- 1/2 cup frozen cranberries
- 1/2 medium frozen banana

DIRECTIONS:

1. In a blender, put in all the ingredients. Puree until smooth in texture. Serve.

Nutrition:
Calories: 245 | Carbohydrates: 50.4 g
Fat: 1.3 g | Protein: 12.5 g

5. PEACH RASPBERRY PUFF PANCAKE

Prep Time: 15 minutes
Cook Time: 20 minutes
Serving Size: 1 pancake slice, 1 tablespoon yogurt, and 1/2 cup fruit

INGREDIENTS:

- 1/2 cup fresh raspberries
- 1/4 cup vanilla yogurt
- 1/2 cup milk (fat-free)
- 1/2 cup all-purpose flour
- 2 medium peaches (peeled, sliced)
- 3 large eggs (room temperature, beaten lightly)
- 1 tablespoon butter
- 1/2 teaspoon sugar
- 1/8 teaspoon salt

DIRECTIONS:

1. Preheat oven to 400 degrees Fahrenheit.
2. In a bowl, toss the peaches and sugar. Stir in gently the raspberries. Set aside.
3. Put the butter on a pie plate. Heat the pie plate in the oven for 3 minutes.
4. In a bowl, whisk well the milk, eggs, and salt. Whisk in the flour gradually.
5. Take out the pie plate from the oven. Spread the melted butter to coat the sides and bottom of the plate. Pour the egg mixture into the pie plate.
6. Bake for 22 minutes. Slice the pancake into 4 parts. Serve with yogurt and fruit mixture.

Nutrition:
Calories: 199 | Carbohydrates: 25 g
Fat: 7 g | Protein: 9 g

6. PEACH TART

Prep Time: 30 minutes
Cook Time: 40 minutes
Serving Size: 1 tart

INGREDIENTS:

- 1 cup all-purpose flour
- 1/4 cup butter (softened)
- 1/4 teaspoon ground nutmeg
- 3 tablespoons sugar

Filling:

- 2 pounds peaches (peeled, sliced)
- 1/4 cup almonds (sliced)
- 1/3 cup sugar
- 1/4 teaspoon ground cinnamon
- 2 tablespoons all-purpose flour
- 1/8 teaspoon almond extract

DIRECTIONS:

1. Preheat oven to 375 degrees Fahrenheit.
2. In a bowl, cream the sugar, nutmeg, and butter until light and fluffy. Beat in the flour.
3. Press the crust firmly on the up sides and bottom of a tart pan.
4. Put on top of a baking sheet. Bake for 12 minutes in the middle rack. Put on the wire rack to cool.
5. In a bowl, put in the sugar, peaches, cinnamon, flour, and almond extract. Toss to combine. Equally portion the tart among the crust. Top with almonds.
6. Bake for 45 minutes on the lower rack. Put them on the wire rack to cool. Serve.

Nutrition:
Calories: 222 | Carbohydrates: 36 g
Fat: 8 g | Protein: 4 g

7. BLUEBERRY APPLE COBBLER

Prep Time: 15 minutes
Cook Time: 40 minutes
Serving Size: 1/8 of the dish

INGREDIENTS:

- 12 ounces fresh blueberries
- 2 large apples (peeled, cored, sliced thinly)
- 2 tablespoons cornstarch
- 2 tablespoons sugar
- 1 tablespoon lemon juice
- 1 teaspoon ground cinnamon

Topping:

- 3/4 cup whole-wheat flour
- 3/4 cup all-purpose flour
- 1/2 cup milk (fat-free)
- 4 tablespoons cold trans-free margarine (cut into pieces)
- 2 tablespoons sugar
- 1 teaspoon vanilla extract
- 1 1/2 teaspoons baking powder
- 1/4 teaspoon salt

DIRECTIONS:

1. Preheat the oven to 400 degrees Fahrenheit. Grease a square baking pan with cooking spray.
2. In a bowl, put in the apple slices. Drizzle with lemon juice.
3. In another bowl, mix well the cinnamon, cornstarch, and sugar. Pour the mixture onto the apple slices. Toss.
4. Mix in the blueberries. Evenly spread the mixture on the greased baking pan. Set aside.
5. In another bowl, mix well the salt, baking powder, sugar, and flours. Mix in the cold margarine pieces into the flour mixture with a fork.
6. Pour in the vanilla and milk. Stir well to form into dough.
7. Gently knead the dough until smooth. Roll the dough with a rolling pin into a 1/2-inch thick rectangle.
8. Cut out shapes using a cookie cutter. Roll out the scraps to make more shapes.

9. Arrange the cut out pieces on top of the blueberry-apple mixture until fully covered.
10. Bake for 30 minutes. Serve.

Nutrition:
Calories: 222 | Carbohydrates: 38 g
Fat: 6 g | Protein: 4 g

8. ORANGE SMOOTHIE

Prep Time: 5 minutes
Cook Time: 0 minutes
Serving Size: 1 cup

INGREDIENTS:

- 1 cup light vanilla soy milk (chilled)
- 1 1/2 cups orange juice (chilled)
- 1/3 cup soft tofu
- 1 teaspoon orange zest (grated)
- 1 tablespoon dark honey
- 5 ice cubes
- 1/2 teaspoon vanilla extract
- 4 peeled orange segments

DIRECTIONS:

1. In a blender, put in the soy milk, orange juice, honey, tofu, vanilla, orange zest, and ice cubes. Blend until frothy.
2. Serve in chilled glasses. Garnish with an orange segment on each glass.

Nutrition:
Calories: 101 | Carbohydrates: 20 g
Fat: 1 g | Protein: 3 g

9. GRILLED ANGEL FOOD CAKE

Prep Time: 10 minutes
Cook Time: 15 minutes
Serving Size: 1 slice with topping

INGREDIENTS:

- 1/2 cup sugar
- 1 1/2 cup strawberries (chopped)
- 3/4 cup low-fat whipped cream (for topping)
- 3/4 cup rhubarb (chopped)
- 6 tablespoons water
- 1/8 teaspoon cinnamon
- 1 3/4 teaspoons vanilla
- 1 prepared angel food cake (6 slices)

DIRECTIONS:

1. Heat the gas grill. Grease the grill rack with cooking spray. Put the grill rack 6 inches above the heat source.
2. In a saucepan over medium heat, mix well the rhubarb, strawberries, water, sugar, cinnamon, and vanilla. Cook for 5 minutes. Turn off the heat. Set aside.
3. Put the cake slices on the edge of the grill rack where the heat is minimal. Grill all sides of the cake slices until browned.
4. Transfer each cake slice on a plate. Top each cake with 1/4 cup of the strawberry mixture and 2 tablespoons of whipped cream. Serve.

Nutrition:
Calories: 169 | Carbohydrates: 38 g
Fat: 1 g | Protein: 2 g

10. CREAM AND COOKIES SHAKE

Prep Time: 5 minutes
Cook Time: 0 minutes
Serving Size: 1 cup

INGREDIENTS:

- 3 cups vanilla ice cream (fat-free)
- 1 1/3 cups vanilla soy milk (chilled)
- 6 chocolate wafer cookies (crushed)

DIRECTIONS:

1. In a blender, put in the ice cream and soy milk. Blend until frothy.
2. Add in the cookies. Pulse to mix well.
3. Pour into chilled glasses. Serve.

Nutrition:
Calories: 270 | Carbohydrates: 52 g
Fat: 3 g | Protein: 9 g

CHAPTER 4:

DASH SNACKS

1. STEAMED ASPARAGUS WITH HORSERADISH DIP

Prep Time: 5 minutes
Cook Time: 15 minutes
Serving Size: 2 asparagus spears and 1 tablespoon dip

INGREDIENTS:

- 32 fresh asparagus spears (trimmed)
- 1/4 cup Parmesan cheese (grated)
- 1 cup mayonnaise (reduced-fat)
- 1/2 teaspoon Worcestershire sauce
- 1 tablespoon prepared horseradish

DIRECTIONS:

1. Place the asparagus in a steamer. Steam for 4 minutes. Immediately transfer the asparagus in ice water. Drain. Pat with paper towels to dry.
2. In a bowl, mix together the rest of the ingredients.
3. Serve the asparagus with the dip.

Nutrition:
Calories: 63 | Carbohydrates: 3 g
Fat: 5 g | Protein: 1 g

2. MINT, LIME, AND GRAPEFRUIT YOGURT PARFAIT

Prep Time: 15 minutes
Cook Time: 0 minutes
Serving Size: 1 parfait glass

INGREDIENTS:

- 4 cups reduced-fat plain yogurt
- 4 large red grapefruit
- 3 tablespoons honey
- 2 tablespoons lime juice
- 2 teaspoons lime zest (grated)
- Fresh mint leaves (torn)

DIRECTIONS:

1. Cut off the peel the grapefruit including the outer membrane. Slice following the membrane on each segment to remove the fruit inside.
2. In a bowl, mix well the lime zest, yogurt, and lime juice. Layer into 6 parfait glasses the half of the grapefruit. The next layer is the half of the yogurt mixture. Repeat the layers.
3. Top each parfait glass with honey and mint. Serve.

Nutrition:
Calories: 207 | Carbohydrates: 39 g
Fat: 3 g | Protein: 10 g

...PS WITH HUMMUS DIP

...minutes
Cook Time: 0 minutes
Serving Size: 1/12 of the dish

INGREDIENTS:

- 1 10-ounce carton hummus
- 1 cup feta cheese (crumbled)
- 1/2 cup Greek olives (chopped)
- 1/4 cup red onion (finely chopped)
- 1 large English cucumber (chopped)
- 2 medium tomatoes (seeded, chopped)
- Baked pita chips

DIRECTIONS:

1. In a shallow round dish, spread the hummus evenly. Layer with onion, tomatoes, olives, cucumber, and cheese.
2. Chill in the fridge for an hour or more. Serve with chips.

Nutrition:
Calories: 88 | Carbohydrates: 6 g
Fat: 5 g | Protein: 4 g

4. ALMOND AND FRUIT BITES

Prep Time: 40 minutes + chilling
Cook Time: 0 minutes
Serving Size: 1 bite

INGREDIENTS:

- 3 3/4 cups sliced almonds (divided)
- 2 cups dried apricots (finely chopped)
- 1 cup pistachios (finely chopped, toasted)
- 1 cup dried cherries (finely chopped)
- 1/4 cup honey
- 1/4 teaspoon almond extract

DIRECTIONS:

1. In a food processor, pulse the 1 1/4 cups of almonds until chopped finely. Transfer to a shallow bowl for coating later.
2. Put in the rest of the almonds into the food processor. Pulse until chopped finely. Add in the almond extract.
3. While pulsing, add the honey gradually. Transfer to a bowl. Stir in the cherries and apricots.
4. Divide the dough into 6 parts. Roll each part into 1/2-inch thick logs. Wrap each log in plastic. Chill in the fridge for an hour to firm.
5. Unwrap each log. Slice into 1 1/2-inch pieces. Roll half of the bites in pistachios. Roll the other half in almonds.
6. Serve or store in airtight containers.

Nutrition:
Calories: 86 | Carbohydrates: 10 g
Fat: 5 g | Protein: 2 g

5. BANANA SPLIT—DASH DIET STYLE

Prep Time: 10 minutes
Cook Time: 0 minutes
Serving Size: 1/4 of the dish

INGREDIENTS:

- 4 small bananas (peeled, halved lengthwise)
- 1 cup fresh raspberries
- 2 cups fat-free vanilla Greek yogurt
- 1/2 cup granola without raisins
- 2 small peaches (sliced)
- 2 tablespoons sunflower kernels
- 2 tablespoons sliced almonds (toasted)
- 2 tablespoons honey

DIRECTIONS:

1. Equally portion the bananas among 4 dishes. Top with the rest of the ingredients. Serve.

Nutrition:
Calories: 340 | Carbohydrates: 61 g
Fat: 6 g | Protein: 17 g

6. CHAI ALMOND GRANOLA

Prep Time: 20 minutes
Cook Time: 1 1/4 hours
Serving Size: 1/2 cup

INGREDIENTS:

- 3 cups quick-cooking oats
- 1 cup shredded coconut (sweetened)
- 2 cups almonds (coarsely chopped)
- 1/2 cup honey
- 1/3 cup sugar
- 1/4 cup boiling water
- 1/4 cup olive oil
- 2 chai tea bags
- 2 teaspoons vanilla extract
- 3/4 teaspoon ground cinnamon
- 3/4 teaspoon salt
- 1/4 teaspoon ground cardamom
- 3/4 teaspoon ground nutmeg

DIRECTIONS:

1. Preheat oven to 250 degrees Fahrenheit. Grease a rimmed baking pan.
2. Steep the tea bags for 5 minutes in boiling water.
3. In a bowl, mix well the coconut, almonds, and oats.
4. Discard the tea bags. Mix well the rest of the ingredients into the tea. Pour the tea mixture into the oat mixture. Mix well.
5. Spread out the mixture evenly on the greased baking pan.
6. Bake for 1 1/4 hours, stirring every 20 minutes.
7. Cool completely. Serve or store in an airtight container.

Nutrition:
Calories: 272 | Carbohydrates: 29 g
Fat: 16 g | Protein: 6 g

7. ALMOND BUTTER AND CHOCOLATE BITES

Prep Time: 5 minutes
Cook Time: 0 minutes
Serving Size: 1 teaspoon almond butter and 2 1/4-ounce squares chocolate

INGREDIENTS:

- 4 teaspoons almond butter
- 8 1/4-ounce squares bittersweet chocolate

DIRECTIONS:

1. Spread 1/2 teaspoon of almond butter on each chocolate square. Serve.

Nutrition:
Calories: 79 | Carbohydrates: 9.4 g
Fat: 5.8 g | Protein: 1.2 g

8. HUMMUS AND VEGETABLES SANDWICH

Prep Time: 10 minutes
Cook Time: 0 minutes
Serving Size: 1 sandwich

INGREDIENTS:

- 3 tablespoons hummus
- 2 slices whole-grain bread
- 1/2 cup mixed salad greens
- 1/4 cup carrot (shredded)
- 1/4 cup cucumber (sliced)
- 1/4 avocado (mashed)
- 1/4 medium red bell pepper (sliced)

DIRECTIONS:

1. Spread the hummus on a slice of bread.
2. Spread the avocado on the other slice of bread.
3. Fill the sandwich with the rest of the ingredients.
4. Slice in half. Serve.

Nutrition:
Calories: 325 | Carbohydrates: 39.7 g
Fat: 14.3 g | Protein: 12.8 g

9. BANANA PEANUT BUTTER CINNAMON TOAST

Prep Time: 5 minutes
Cook Time: 0 minutes
Serving Size: 1 toast

INGREDIENTS:

- 1 small banana (sliced)
- 1 tablespoon peanut butter
- 1 slice whole-wheat bread (toasted)
- Cinnamon (to taste)

DIRECTIONS:

1. Spread the peanut butter on the toast. Arrange the banana slices on top.
2. Garnish with cinnamon. Serve.

Nutrition:
Calories: 266 | Carbohydrates: 38.3 g
Fat: 9.3 g | Protein: 8.1 g

10. OAT WITH PEANUT BUTTER ENERGY BALLS

Prep Time: 15 minutes
Cook Time: 15 minutes
Serving Size: 1 energy ball

INGREDIENTS:

- 1/4 cup natural peanut butter
- 1/2 cup rolled oats
- 3/4 cup Medjool dates (chopped)
- Chia seeds (for garnish)

DIRECTIONS:

1. In a bowl with hot water, soak the dates for 10 minutes. Drain.
2. In a food processor, put in the oats, dates, and peanut butter. Process until chopped finely.
3. Roll the mixture into 12 balls. Garnish with chia seeds.
4. Chill in the fridge for an hour or more. Serve.

Nutrition:
Calories: 73 | Carbohydrates: 10.1 g
Fat: 3 g | Protein: 1.8 g

CONCLUSION

Once again, thank you for purchasing this book. It is my hope and pleasure that you have found the DASH diet to be very feasible and easy to apply in your life. I hope that you get started on it as quickly as you can so you can reap the benefits of this diet sooner.

I have always found that this diet is the easiest pathway to better management of hypertension. I hope that you have enjoyed the recipes that I have included as much as I did when I tried them for the first time.

The good news is that there are plenty of DASH diet recipes and you will never run out of options. Remember that my goal in this book is to get you started on this type of diet. If you found that the recipes to be easy, enjoyable to eat, and the diet itself doesn't force you to make a lot of drastic and unrealistic changes in your meals, then it is definitely a diet that can best suit you.

The next step is to find more DASH diet recipes that are best suited for women of all ages. After you have added more recipes in your collection, you should create a meal plan that can last you for several weeks.

Think of all of this as an adventure that involves finding heart healthy food that will help you become a better woman.

I thank you again for traversing through the pages of this book and hope that you will find the DASH diet as a sustainable solution for hypertension.

Manufactured by Amazon.ca
Bolton, ON